Stolen Moments

Stolen Moments

Coping with Loss from Multiple Sclerosis

PAULETTE REN

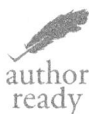

author
ready

For information contact:
authorpauletteren.com
authorpaulette.ren@gmail.com

Published by:
Author Ready

Content Editor: Debbie Ihler Rasmussen • authordebbieihlerrasmussen.com
Copy Editor: Kim Autrey • neveralonepublishing.com

Cover design by Trivuj • 99designs
Interior book design by Francine Platt, Eden Graphics, Inc.
edengraphics.net

Paperback ISBN 978-1-958626-26-9
Ebook ISBN 978-1-958626-27-6

Library of Congress Number: 2022922599

Manufactured in the United States of America

First Edition

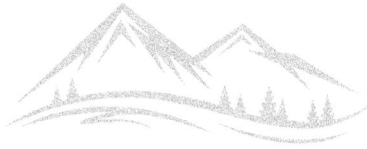

To My Husband—
Not enough time with the
one I love.

Dear Readers,

This is a true story but many of the names were changed to make it easier to write. Any resemblance to actual names, characters and incidents, living or dead, is entirely coincidental.

I hope you enjoy the book and know the main purpose of writing it was to give others suffering from a chronic disease, the hope and encouragement they need to go on. Life is worth living and your attitude and taking care of yourself is so important. Be positive.

Love to all,

PAULETTE REN

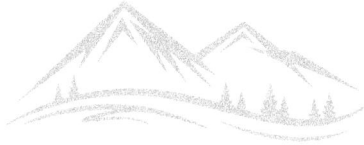

Prologue

I have always been fascinated by time. Have you ever stopped to think about TIME?

You wake up, and before you know it, time for bed. One day goes by, a week, a month, and then a year. There are only 24 hours in a day. It's the same every single day; yet some days seem to whiz by, while others drag.

Why is that?

I have heard it said that when you get older, time goes by more quickly. But that just doesn't make sense.

TIME is TIME, isn't it?

I'm 76 years old and have no idea how I got here so fast. I still feel like a teenager in some ways; although, my body doesn't always agree with that.

I have a story to tell you about time. The main character is my husband of thirty-three years, Antonio Amante Jr.

My name is Natalie Amante, I suppose I am the supporting character because this story isn't only his; it's mine, too. This is our story of stolen moments.

Antonio was diagnosed with multiple sclerosis when he was thirty and lived with the disease the rest of his life.

I wonder what life would have been like if this had not happened. Life is precious; you never know what it will bring. So many stolen moments taught our family to be strong and hopeful with whatever came our way. Moment by moment, day by day, we strived to have faith, hope, and love while doing our best under the circumstances.

Chapter One

Life is not what you expect.
It is made of the most unexpected twists and turns.

− LLAIYARAAJA

I have always felt that things happen for a reason, but I couldn't for the life of me understand why God was being so cruel. I knew this day would come, so why was I so surprised?

I was in pain from the devastation of knowing this was happening to us. How could we go from being so happy and enjoying life, to suddenly so many changes?

It didn't seem fair. We were good people. Good Christian people who were always helping others and yet not wanting to burden others. What would we do now?

I was brought up in the Catholic Church, yet all those years believing in God didn't console me. I was hurt, angry, and didn't want our lives to change.

Accepting our circumstances took me a long time. A very long time.

As I walked the hall to Antonio's hospital room, the smell of antiseptic filled the air. I noticed the nurses sitting around as I reached for the hand sanitizer before entering his room. I didn't want to be there, but Antonio had rapidly deteriorated to his weakest state.

I would rather it be me. My heart ached, and my eyes burned from weeping, but I hid my emotions, walked to Antonio's bedside, kissed his forehead, and sat next to him.

"Hi, Honey, how are you feeling today?"

Our eyes met, and I could see he had been crying, too.

"What do we do now?" his voice cracked.

"We'll do whatever we have to. We'll make you comfortable and continue with our family's life. Between the kids and me, we'll make it work."

"I love you, Natalie." Antonio squeezed my hand.

"I love you, too."

And we both cried.

My sweet husband, Antonio Amante Jr. lay in a hospital bed paralyzed from the neck down. He couldn't move his hands, arms, or legs. He would need complete care to perform normal daily tasks. Showering, shaving, brushing his teeth, dressing, and eating.

He was going blind, only seeing shadows.

Maybe the worst part for Antonio was he still had a sharp mind and voice. He was painfully aware of everything happening around him. He expressed that he felt crushed, defeated, and helpless.

Multiple sclerosis is an incurable disease in which the insulating covers of the nerve cells in the brain and the spinal cord are damaged. He was originally diagnosed when he was thirty years old, and though the effects were ever present, now in his fifties, the disease had progressed to his present condition, lying helpless in a hospital bed.

Antonio knew he could only surrender and let others take care of him. Including me, Natalie, his wife of thirty-three years. His biggest concern was how he was going to take care of his family. After all these years of being together, this disease finally brought all of us to the realization that life would never be the same.

Chapter Two

The love in our family flows strong and deep,
leaving us memories to treasure and keep.
- AUTHOR UNKNOWN

Antonio Amante grew up in Midvale, Utah, a suburb of Salt Lake City, to hard-working Italian parents. Family was of prime importance to them. They were careful with their money, making sure they had food on the table and a roof over their heads. They loved being together.

Antonio was the oldest and his father's namesake. He had two younger brothers, Luca and Thomas.

Antonio Sr. looked like many Italians you might see in the movies. Short and round, he could have easily been mistaken for one of the Mafia guys. A strong man from years of working in the Kennecott Copper Mines with many of his family and friends. Outspoken, and somewhat rough around the edges, he had a great sense of humor making him fun to be around. He told stories and jokes for hours to anyone who would listen, but depending on the situation, he could be grumpy or moody.

Bianca, Antonio's mother, was petite with dark, brown hair. Most of her life she struggled with rheumatoid arthritis, lung, and heart problems, but she never gave in to her weaknesses.

A very caring, emotional person, she helped others whenever she could, and she worked hard to make a happy home for her family. With her amusing sense of humor, Bianca was fun to be around, too.

Painfully frugal, she saved everything. She would wash and reuse plastic bags, tin foil, wrapping paper; anything she could salvage for another time. She loved cooking and managed to have plenty of good food for everyone to enjoy.

When Antonio was a teenager, he took accordion lessons from Larry Pino and soon became part of the Larry Pino Symphonic Accordion Band. They traveled all over the United States for competitions in Colorado, Kansas, Illinois, and more.

His family was so proud of him as he often placed first or at least in the top three.

On his mother's side were an extended family, with several aunts, uncles, and cousins who were very close and loved to spend time together. Holidays, birthdays, weddings, baptisms, anything that was important warranted a celebration.

They all loved to cook deliciously mouthwatering recipes, especially Italian food, and their tables were banquet-worthy, with enough food for an army.

They enjoyed spending time together in nature. Camping, fishing, hunting, hiking, and long weekends at a favorite destination. There was always plenty of food including lumberjack breakfasts of potatoes, ham, bacon, sausage, eggs, fruit, juice, and coffee. Dinners were fabulous and plenty of snacks were readily available.

They rode motorcycles and played games, telling stories into the night around the campfire, often about their ancestors. Laughing and enjoying the moments together, they were a fun group to be around.

Italians love to eat, and I learned quickly if they offered you something, they would be very offended if you turned it down. It was best to just take a little of everything and enjoy the fabulous smell and taste. Over the years, the cooks were named "Food Bullies'" because they wouldn't take no for an answer.

Chapter Three

An intelligent man will open your mind,
a handsome man will open your eyes,
and a gentleman will open your heart.

- AUTHOR UNKNOWN

Antonio's dark, curly hair and deep blue eyes made him a strikingly handsome man, who was very proud of his Italian heritage.

Smaller built than most men, Antonio was around five feet eight inches, weighing about a hundred fifty pounds. His weight rarely fluctuated more than five pounds during his lifetime. He must have had a good metabolism, because he loved to eat, especially when his mom or Nonna (grandma) were doing the cooking.

Friends often told him he looked like Errol Flynn, an actor from the nineteen thirties and forties. Today, he might be compared to Al Pacino or Robert DeNiro. Family, friends, and even strangers commented on his good looks, but he didn't see himself like others did.

Antonio loved nice clothes, often wearing Gant shirts that were popular at the time, with a nice ascot tie and dress slacks. He was a classy guy.

He loved fast expensive cars. Over the years, he was the proud owner of an Austin Healey, Pontiac GTO, Mercedes, and Lincoln, to name a few.

He loved good liquor, especially Scotch and Crown Royal. He would sip on his drink, listen to music, mostly jazz, and smoke his pipe while reading *Playboy* magazine (you know, for the articles).

Antonio admired a certain class of men; successful, rich, and knew what they wanted. He was smart, logical, frugal, and set many goals. He wanted to be a millionaire by the time he was thirty, so he read articles, newsletters, magazines, and kept up on any information that would help him attain his dreams.

Before Antonio's illness took so much away from him, he was extremely active and enjoyed the outdoors. He loved the mountains of Utah and spent many days enjoying his passions of snow skiing, boating, water skiing, golfing, and hiking.

Chapter Four

He stirred my soul in the most subtle way and
the story between us wrote itself.

—NIKKI ROWE

Antonio and I crossed paths in an unusual way, but
I have no doubt destiny played a major role.

I have always been a firm believer that things are
meant to be and happen for a reason. My family
often questioned my beliefs, but esoteric subjects and
the unknown always fascinated me. Why do things
happen as they do? Sometimes, there is no clear or
logical answer, and this is how I felt about mine and
Antonio's chance meeting.

In 1966, Antonio was working for an engineering firm who did contract work for various states.
His company wanted him to move to Pocatello,
Idaho, to work on a special project for a company
called Food Machinery Company (FMC). They
needed a designer for various machines and furnaces;

Antonio's expertise as a draftsman was a perfect fit. The job was scheduled to take six months to a year to complete, and Antonio decided this would be good for him financially and for the experience he would gain. He was close enough to his home in Utah that he could go back on weekends and enjoy his hobbies and spend time with his family.

Antonio found an apartment in a complex where a dear friend of mine and her husband lived. Faye and her husband Jim were expecting their first child.

Faye and Antonio became acquainted while doing their weekly laundry in the shared laundry room of the apartments. They chatted about their lives, and Faye found out that Antonio was single.

"I have several friends who are single," Faye told him. "I could line you up if you decide to date while living in Pocatello."

Antonio raised his eyebrows. "I'm seeing a girl in Utah, but nothing serious."

"Well, let me know if you decide you are interested." Faye smiled at him. "My friends are cute and fun to be around."

"I'll think about that."

Antonio lived in a basement apartment, and Faye and Jim were on the first floor above him.

One day, I went to visit Faye to see how she was doing with her pregnancy and married life. When I first arrived, just as I got to the bottom of the stairs, Antonio came out of his apartment.

Surprised, I said, "Hello," and proceeded up the stairs. I had never seen him before, but he was cute, and I wondered who he was.

I visited with Faye for an hour or so.

Antonio must have been watching because as soon as I left, he knocked on Faye's door.

"Who was that girl that just came to see you? Is she one of your friends you were telling me about?"

"Yes. Her name is Natalie."

He didn't hesitate. "She is gorgeous with killer legs. She's the one I want to meet."

Faye called me to see if it was all right to give Antonio my phone number, and I agreed. A few days later, Antonio called to ask me out to dinner.

Our attraction to each other was instant. Our first date we talked about anything and everything discovering we had a lot in common, including some of the same goals.

We were both Catholic, so we already had many of the same values ingrained in us from our upbringing. We both wanted to be married someday and have children. Family was important to both of us, and we wanted to have good, solid family relationships.

Chapter Five

Anyone who falls in love
is searching for the missing pieces of themselves.

—AUTHOR UNKNOWN

It was August when Antonio and I met. I was preparing to go back to Idaho State University, and Antonio was nearly finished with his studies at the University of Utah. He decided he would put them on hold since he had gotten such a good job with the engineering company. The project in Pocatello was very lucrative, so that made his decision easy.

When we met, my daughter, Adrienne, was a year old. Her father was not in the picture, so I was raising her alone with the help of my parents. I told Antonio about her immediately, I didn't want things to be uncomfortable.

I told him I would totally understand if he chose not to pursue me because I had a child, but to my delight, it didn't seem to bother him. I was so relieved.

At that time in my life, Adrienne was my primary concern. I hoped to find a father for her and have a solid family, but if it didn't work for Antonio, I was fine with that.

At the beginning of our courtship, Antonio would spend time with me during the week, and then go home to Utah on the weekends. It wasn't long before we became inseparable and spent all our free time together.

Antonio was different than most men I had known, and I fell in love. He had goals, knew what he wanted in life, and he was mature and focused.

He was so kind to Adrienne. He would invite us over and cook dinner for us, and we would get together often after work to listen to music and talk. We both loved all kinds of music, especially jazz.

Antonio knew I enjoyed sewing, and one Sunday when he stayed in town, he asked, "Would you bring over your sewing machine and do some mending for me?"

"Sure," I happily agreed.

"I'll cook dinner in exchange."

"Sounds good to me."

I don't think mending is much of a thing any-more, but it was normal back then.

And so, it went—we were like a domestic family. We stayed home during the day doing chores, and

Adrienne running around the apartment playing with toys I brought over to Antonio's for her.

One day, there was a knock on the door. Antonio was in another room busy with something, so I went to answer it with Adrienne following me.

A woman asked for Antonio, noticing Adrienne next to me. Embarrassed, I went to find him and let him know someone was at the door to see him. He went outside to talk to her. Apparently, it was Norma, his girlfriend from Utah. Since he was spending more time in Idaho, she had decided she would come there to see him.

He broke up with her that day and let her know he was falling in love with me. I felt bad for Norma, and I was sorry she found out this way, but what is that old saying? "All is fair in love and war."

We had been seeing each other for about a month when Antonio's grandfather, (Nonno) became ill. Antonio was very close to him and had spent much of his growing years with his Nonna and Nonno. He loved them so much. They were always so happy when he went to visit them. He helped them when he could, and they always cooked his favorite Italian meals for him when he visited. Some of his favorites were gnocchi, buttered pasta, polenta with chicken stew, lasagna, and spaghetti.

His grandfather died before the month was over,

and Antonio was devastated. He stayed in Utah for a week to be with his family during this sad time. After the funeral, Antonio returned to Idaho and went back to work.

Antonio was down about his grandfather's death, and he talked a lot about his childhood and his closeness to his family. His sorrow and vulnerability brought us even closer together. I just wanted to hold him and comfort him and let him know, in time, it would all be okay. One can never forget the sorrow of a loss, but time helps us to heal. After a while, it can become easier to talk about the deceased and remember all the good times you shared.

Chapter Six

*Having somewhere to go is home. Having someone
to love is family and having both is a blessing.*

—AUTHOR UNKNOWN

By December, Antonio and I were *an item*; not
dating anyone else. We were beginning to talk
about marriage.

He asked me to go to Salt Lake for his company's Christmas party, and while there, he planned
to introduce me to his parents and friends. Antonio
had told me so much about all of them. I was nervous, but it was time to get to know them and see
how they reacted to me.

We arrived in Salt Lake in the afternoon and went
directly to his parents' house. His father was outside
puttering around in the garden area of the yard. First
thing out of his mouth was, "Are you guys going to
get married or what?"

I felt my face turn bright red, but I didn't say a word.

His dad scared me. He was stocky, looked strong, with a deep loud voice. Antonio just laughed and introduced us, then he took me into the house to meet his mother, Bianca.

She was very sweet and friendly. "I'm so happy to meet you, Natalie. We've heard so much about you. Would you like something to drink?"

"No thank you. I'm happy to meet you, too."

She kept asking, then finally, Antonio told her I liked milk. How was I to know that eating and drinking was a big thing for the Italians? They were easily offended by turning them down when offered something to eat.

I learned that fast.

Antonio had two brothers, Luca and Thomas, who were several years younger than him. I didn't meet either of them that first time. Luca was at college in Southern Utah, and Thomas was in high school.

The company Christmas party was so much fun. We got all dressed up and spent the night meeting all his work buddies and their partners. We ate, danced, and drank a lot. They were kind to me and happy to see Antonio had found someone special. They seemed to be a great bunch of people who liked to enjoy life.

I was so glad to mix with this group. This life was all new to me and seemed so exciting. Even though I had good friends in Pocatello, I had never gone to many activities like this party. It was so nice to get all fancy and enjoy the night.

After the holidays, Antonio and I talked seriously about getting married. We wanted to set a date but decided it would be best to talk to our parents and let them know our intentions.

My family was very poor and didn't have a lot of extra money. Dad always worked two jobs to provide for Mom and us nine kids.

Dad worked at the Union Pacific Railroad and another job at a bar where he oversaw the card room where patrons mostly played poker. Just surviving was difficult.

My parents liked Antonio and seemed open to our plans of marriage. After speaking to them, they said they could possibly help if it was in June or after, but most of the expenses would have to be on Antonio and me.

I worked for a car dealership at the time, so my goal was to save a little money from each paycheck toward the wedding.

While we were making wedding plans, Antonio's engineering firm asked him if he would be willing to go to Fullerton, California, and open an office there. They wanted it done before summer.

Antonio didn't want to go without me, so we decided on an April wedding, even though we knew most of the expenses were on us. With only about three months to plan the wedding, it was a hectic time.

We set the date of April 15, 1967, only eight months after we met. I often teased Antonio he chose that date so he would have a tax write-off.

To save money, I decided to make my own wedding dress and the bridesmaid dresses. Mom and I drove to Salt Lake to look for material where larger fabric stores would offer more choices than our small town like Pocatello.

I found a beautiful Italian lace, perfect for my dress, then netting and accessories to make my veil.

I wanted happy, bright colors for the bridesmaids. I found a lovely fabric, with big yellow flowers on it. Looking back now I wondered what I was thinking as it was so bold! But it was appropriate for the 1960's. Our wedding would be in the afternoon, so I wanted it to look like a tea party with bridesmaids wearing hats.

Chapter Seven

For it was not into my ear you whispered, but into my heart. It was not my lips you kissed, but my soul.

—JUDY GARLAND

My dress was simple with a round neck and emphasizing the beautiful lace. Three-quarter-length sleeves with yellow, satin lining matched the color scheme in the tea-length dress. My grandmother helped me by hand stitching white, pearl buttons down the back. I wore a single, pearl necklace with pearl earrings to match.

I fashioned my veil with an on-the-forehead headpiece of organdy centered with pearls to hold my bouffant style netting. Antonio's grandmother had made a beautiful lace handkerchief especially for this occasion. I held it with my flower bouquet.

Everything for the wedding was coming together as planned. But one important thing I wanted do before we got married was for Antonio to adopt

Adrienne. We had all the necessary paperwork and needed to show we were to be married in the Catholic Church. Since we were moving to California after the wedding, the judge set the court date for the adoption before our wedding.

We took Adrienne with us that day, and I was so happy looking forward to our life together. Antonio was a good man, and I felt lucky to have found him. We looked into each other's eyes as tears flowed from both of us. It was a such a heartfelt and touching moment for both of us.

Our wedding took place in the beautiful church where I grew up. St. Anthony's Parish. It was a very traditional church with mass spoken in Italian. Colorful, stained-glass windows portrayed biblical stories and enormous statues of St. Anthony, St. Joseph, the Virgin Mary, and other saints were displayed in the front and back of the church. A large statue of Jesus on the cross hung on the wall where the altar was. Candles were available in the back of the church for those people who wanted to light one and say a prayer. A common practice in the Catholic Church, prayers were often said for those who were suffering, ill, or in need of help. The priests and nuns who ran the church were very strict, but I loved the church itself.

Common to Catholic weddings, we had a nuptial

mass at noon. If both members of the wedding couple are Catholic, they can have a full Catholic ceremony. The nuptial mass includes additional readings from the Old and New Testaments.

One of Antonio's aunts owned a floral shop in Utah and made the flowers for us. Two beautiful altar bouquets of chrysanthemums, roses, and lilies. My bouquet of gardenias, orchids, and yellow roses in a cascade style, accented with streamers of yellow ribbon.

My friend Pam served as my maid of honor, and Faye was a bridesmaid. Two of my sisters, Sage and Lulu, were junior bridesmaids. Their identical street-length dresses were yellow and orange floral. They wore yellow shoes, white gloves, and white brimmed hats. Their flower bouquets were yellow chrysanthemums with green leaves and green ribbon streamers.

Luca, Antonio's brother, performed the best man duties, and Keith, one of my brothers, was a bridegroom. My sister Lilly sat at the guest book.

My dad held my hand as we stood in the back of the church waiting for the ceremony to begin. I was nervous and embarrassed to think all these people would be looking at me.

The altar looked a mile away.

I took a few deep breaths as the organ began to play, our cue to march down the aisle.

In the middle of the ceremony, I placed a bouquet

of flowers at the feet of the Virgin Mary statue. I said a prayer and thanked her for helping me find such a good man and asked her to bless our marriage.

The wedding ceremony was solemn and serious but beautiful and touching. It was perfect. I would remember this day forever.

Immediately following the wedding, we went downstairs for a reception. My grandmother had made lace tablecloths for the serving tables. Cake, coffee, and punch were served by my two good friends, Janice and Susan. I think every relative of Antonio's came for the wedding. I felt sad we didn't have food served for those coming from out of town, but the cake and drinks were all we could afford.

Afterward, our parents, families, and some of our relatives did go over to my grandmother's house for a small luncheon.

The very next day, we headed to Utah for a reception there that was put on by Antonio's parents and relatives. His mother, grandmother, aunts, and their families had been baking, cooking, and preparing for this event for days. I had never seen so much food. It was an Italian feast with everything you could imagine.

Platters of salami, ham, roast beef, turkey, and all the trimmings. Homemade rolls, potato, macaroni, frogeye, and green salads in beautiful bowls. One aunt had made a wedding cake and baked dozens of Greek almond cookies. Other family members made pound cakes, banana breads, zucchini breads, and lots of assorted cookies. So many delicious trays of food with wine flowing freely. Everything was prepared so beautifully, and the food was delicious.

Most of his relatives and friends attended, so I met many of the people Antonio had told me stories about. Between the Pocatello and Utah receptions, we received lots of gifts and money to start our lives together. It was amazing, and I was so grateful to everyone for doing so much for us. Our married journey was beginning, and what a wonderful way to start.

Chapter Eight

Life is a relentless exploration in search of happiness.
—AUTHOR UNKNOWN

Antonio bought a new 1967 white Pontiac GTO before we left for California to open the new office. After all the wedding hoopla was over, we loaded the car to the hilt and headed for our new home. Excitement can't begin to describe my enthusiasm. I had a new husband, new car, beautiful apartment, and moving to a new state to begin a new life.

I had done very little traveling, and this adventure was an answer to my prayers. We stopped in Las Vegas for the night; had never been there before. The city was such a bustling, interesting place. I hoped we could come back again as there was so much to see. Over the years, Las Vegas became one of our favorite destinations.

The next morning, we had breakfast and headed for our new home in Fullerton, California. Adrienne was so excited to be going on a trip even though she didn't know where we were going. She probably thought it was a fun adventure.

Our apartment was in a very secluded area on a cul-de-sac. Parking was underground, and it appeared safe. The grounds were immaculately maintained as well as the pool. We were looking forward to spending a lot of time in the warm sunshine.

The complex was new, so everything was modern and up-to-date. Our apartment had two bedrooms and two baths. To me, it was so perfect. I was anxious to decorate, to put our signature on our new home. Gratefulness filled my heart.

Over the next week, we got settled, put our gifts and other belongings away, and Antonio started back to work. I started planning domestic life as a new wife.

I was a fanatic for cleaning and organization, so I started a weekly schedule to get all chores done. A daily, written menu of everything I planned to do; cleaning, grocery shopping, preparing meals, laundry, and ironing. I had dinner on the table every night when Antonio got home from work. I liked to cook, and over the years, I had helped my mother and grandmother prepare meals. I loved to get new recipes and put considerable effort into making delicious dishes.

I wanted to make Antonio happy.

Adrienne and I both enjoyed our time at home, and somedays when all chores were done, we would go to the pool. She loved it, and I was always a sun lover, so I would lay out and get tan. She was a happy child, and I was a happy wife and mother.

On weekends when Antonio was off, we explored California. We often went to different beaches. Laguna, Huntington, Newport, and others. We went to a different one each time and often went to the flea market. We looked for furniture, home décor, and things we needed for the apartment. It was fascinating to see all the interesting places and endless variety of items you could find all over Orange County and the Los Angeles area.

In the 1960's, there was competition to get your business, so many banks would offer gifts if you opened an account with them. When we opened an account near us, we received a beautiful set of stoneware dishes that we used for many years. We found lots of fun surprises living there. It was so different from living in Idaho and not having those perks.

We would get together with guys and their wives from work on the weekends. Antonio and some of his friends had bought a membership to the Playboy Club in Los Angeles. About once a month, we would go there for dinner and entertainment. The food, drinks, and service were excellent. The Playboy Playmates were just as beautiful and shapely as you would expect them to be. I had always thought maybe they were touched up in the magazines to make them look good, but after seeing them live, I was amazed how stunning they really were. We had some fun times there.

Antonio and I were both enjoying married life and learning about each other. We were happy, but then I got sick and ended up in the hospital. The doctor said I had *Honeymoon Cystitis,* a urinary tract infection that many newlyweds get from too much sex. Unfortunately, the infection had backed up into my kidneys and caused some damage to one kidney. The doctor put me on antibiotics, but it took me time to get feeling better and regain my energy. I worried that part of my fatigue was caused by coming from an elevation in Idaho of 4000 to 5000 feet to sea level. I was tired all the time and had to push myself to get things done. Gratefully, eventually my health improved. I didn't want to start having health problems.

Chapter Nine

Sometimes the best thing that you can do
is not think, not wonder, not imagine, not obsess.
Just BREATHE and have faith that everything
will work out for the best.

—AUTHOR UNKNOWN

The next few months we just enjoyed each other and married life, and I always looked forward to Antonio getting home from work.

He was in Army Reserves, and in the summer would go to annual training for two weeks. We decided it would be an ideal time to have some of my family come to stay with me. My sisters, Sage and Lulu would be coming, and I was so excited! Sage was thirteen, and Lulu fourteen; they hadn't traveled much, so we made big plans. I wanted to make it special, to take them to Knotts Berry Farm, Disneyland, and our favorite beaches.

We got everything ready the night before Sage and Lulu's train was to arrive.

Sometime in the early morning, maybe two or three o'clock, the sound of honking woke me up. I thought it was just people partying or coming home from the bars, but the noise continued, and I couldn't go back to sleep. We were to pick the girls up at the train station at five o'clock.

Suddenly, someone pounded on our front door yelling that there was a fire in the underground parking, and we needed to evacuate.

We had read in the newspaper that an arsonist was going around the Los Angeles area burning cars. Apparently, he would call the police and tell them he was hitting that night, but they never knew where he would be. It was freaky and scary!

Our apartment manager had been suspicious the arsonist might hit our complex, so he put a cot in the parking garage and had been sleeping there for about a week.

On the night of the fire, the manager went back to his apartment to use the bathroom and get a snack. The arsonist must have been watching, and as soon as the manager left, the arsonist ran into the garage and doused several cars with gas, then started them on fire. He escaped before the manager got back.

All the residents, including us, stood around in

shock watching the fire and smoke flow out the parking garage. It took a long time to get the fire under control once the fire department arrived, so it was hours before we knew which cars were burned.

With no cell phones, we had no way of contacting my sisters. We tried to call the small train station, but typically, they locked up after the train arrived, so they didn't answer.

We found out later that Sage and Lulu were put out of the station, with their luggage locked inside. When they didn't see us, they were scared to death. They were in a foreign place with no one around.

They found a pay phone and tried to call us, but since we had been evacuated, we were outside and not able to answer.

When we realized we weren't going to be able to get to our car, Antonio borrowed the manager's home phone and called Jim at his work and asked if we could borrow his car to pick up my sisters.

It was nearly eight o'clock in the morning when we finally made it, and my sisters were terrified.

Sobbing, I jumped out of the car, ran to them, and pulled them both into a tight hug. I apologized for putting them in such a scary situation, especially since they were teenagers. I felt terrible about it.

When we got back to our apartment building, we learned that eight cars had been destroyed. A gas can was left on the hood of our car, so the police figured ours was the last to be hit.

The apartments were severely damaged by the smoke. The carpets, walls, drapes, and nearly everything had to be cleaned in most of the units.

I was only twenty-one, and the legal age to rent a car was twenty-five, so there we were. Antonio was leaving on Monday, and we had no car. The fun vacation we had planned for my sisters was about to change.

I was upset, and Antonio was worried about his car, but there wasn't much we could do. It was a disaster!

When we got back to the apartment, Antonio tried to make it fun for them, so he started a water fight in our backyard. He was trying to make light of the dismal beginning of their vacation. I wasn't in the best of moods after the whole ordeal. I had spent days cleaning the glass on the patio door, and it was shining.

Antonio, Sage, and Lulu were getting water everywhere. My OCD set in, and I lost it. They were making such a mess, and I was tired after spending so much time cleaning the week before.

I went outside and yelled, "Enough already! You guys have really screwed up my nice clean window."

"Oh, Natalie, chill out, we were just having a little fun," said Antonio.

Paulette Ren

"We'll help you clean it up," said Sage

Lulu agreed. "We're sorry, Natalie."

Antonio left on Monday, so the girls and I spent several days tanning, swimming, and enjoying the pool. Adrienne loved the water, so it was fun for her, too.

One day when we left the pool, Sage was leading the way and went through the gate first. Suddenly, she screamed, and then we all screamed.

There was a giant tarantula spider on the gate. It scared us because none of us had ever seen one before. We hurried to report it to the manager. Apparently, the fire had sent many little creatures outside.

We were afraid to go back to the pool after that, so the rest of the week we did manicures and pedicures on each other.

The tarantula was the first thing, starting one mishap after another. Sage spilled some polish on our new table, leaving a big mark. Next, Lulu was ironing, dropped the iron on the new carpet burning a perfect shape of the hot appliance.

Things were not going well, and I became disillusioned and disappointed in how life was changing.

One day, my friend Arlene called to see if she could take us all to the beach to get us out of the house. What a blessing! Just what we needed. She picked up me, my sisters, and Adrienne, and they played in the water and with Arlene's daughter for hours. It was such a great day and perfect to put us in a better mood.

Antonio got home and found a car to use until we could get a new one. He took us to Knotts Berry Farm, SeaWorld, and the beach. We didn't make it to Disneyland but had fun and made up for the past two weeks of disappointment. I had enjoyed having my sisters with us but felt bad that everything had been so mixed up.

I cried when they left for home. I loved them and missed them. I hoped next time would be a better experience. When I looked back on it, what a strange couple of weeks it had been. What started out as an exciting journey to California soon became a nightmare.

First, I got sick, then I ended up in the hospital. Then the arsonist burned our brand-new car, the minor incidents of the table, and Lulu burning the carpet. It seemed like our life was unraveling before us and all in just a matter of about three months since we moved to California.

Chapter Ten

Life is a journey for us all. We all face trials.
We all have ups and downs. All of us are human,
but we are also masters of our fate. We are the ones
who decide how we are going to react to life.

—ELIZABETH SMART

One weekend in the summer, Antonio's friend Tom and his girlfriend invited us to go to Lake Mead. Tom had a nice boat, and we decided to go spend a few days in the sunshine, boating and having fun. We made reservations for the weekend looking forward to water skiing, drinking, and having a blast. Antonio had really missed his favorite sports. Since leaving Utah, he hadn't been able to do any of them.

I even tried waterskiing, even though I wasn't very good. I was fearful and had a hard time relaxing. I figured if I didn't learn some of the things Antonio loved, I would be alone on weekends. So,

I ventured out of my comfort zone and did my best to participate.

At night, the complex we were staying at had an area for bonfires. We roasted hot dogs, made smores, drank, laughed, and told jokes and stories.

At some point, I said something naughty. I don't remember what it was. Antonio walked over to me and slapped me across the face. "Don't talk like that," he said.

I was shocked! I had never seen this side of him. Was he jealous? Was it a powerplay in front of his friends? I looked him in the eyes, fury took over, and I snapped. "Don't you ever touch me again, or I will be gone."

Antonio's friends became quiet; they probably didn't know what to say.

I left and went back to our room.

Growing up, I had witnessed too many confrontations between my parents. Watching that caused a hurt so deep that I swore I would never allow a man to treat me like that.

Antonio and I didn't speak the rest of the night or the next day. All the way home, there was a cold silence, and I felt bad our friends had to witness it. I was hurt and embarrassed, and I couldn't believe what he had done. I'd never seen Antonio behave like that.

After returning home, I stayed mad at him for days, and he never apologized. What didn't I know about this man I married? Had I missed something in him? He was always so kind. I knew he was jealous of other men. Was it because I came from a poor family and a small town?

I never did get an answer. Antonio never hit me again in the thirty-three years we were married.

We had to find another car after the fire, and since our car was totaled, the insurance company paid for a replacement. Antonio was so mad about his GTO getting burned that he wasn't about to buy another new one, so we spent some time looking for a used car. We found a used blue Buick Riviera that was in good condition and just a few years old.

We ended up staying in California for only about a year. Once the office was up and running smoothly, Antonio had the chance to move back to Utah. He missed his family and his sports, so we moved back. We stayed with his grandmother for about three months while looking for a house.

Nonna was lonely, and she adored Adrienne, so she loved having us there. Petite, sweet, and kind, she taught me to cook by sharing secret sauces of great Italian cooking. I cooked while she supervised, so that I could learn. I grew to love her very much and appreciated not only her lessons in cooking but all that she did for us.

Antonio wanted me to join him in skiing, so our first Christmas, he bought me skis, boots, and a ski outfit, and I enrolled in Brighton Ski school. I was nervous and afraid. I had never participated much in sports growing up. After my lessons, I felt comfortable enough, but never got over my fear. I was afraid I would break a leg, or someone would run into me.

Nonna and Antonio's mother were happy to watch Adrienne for us while we went skiing once a week during the season. We were fortunate on those days to come home to a big weekend dinner that was always delicious. Italians love to have family dinners, especially on the weekends when most of the family were off work. Nonna and Bianca would take turns watching Adrienne and preparing the dinners. I felt so happy they took both Adrienne and me in and accepted us as family. They were always good to us.

Chapter Eleven

A new home is more than just a house.
It's a present and future with no boundaries.

—AUTHOR UNKNOWN

Antonio and I found a cute house in the Olympus Hills area of Salt Lake City. The house was a great starter home with two bedrooms, two baths, and an unfinished basement. The best part of the house was the yard. In the back was a swimming pool, and the yard was beautifully landscaped with various bushes and roses amongst a variety of perennial flowers. We had an amazing view of Mt. Olympus from the backyard.

The yard proved to be a lot of work to keep up, but we were young and enjoyed the fact that this was our house. As I remember, we paid about $21,000 for the house. We were nervous about having a mortgage and worried if we could pay for it all, but real estate was a good investment, and we had to start somewhere.

On Mother's Day, Antonio bought me golf clubs and lessons, so I could learn another one of his favorite hobbies. He was passionate about golf. I found it to be a fun sport, and I wasn't afraid to play. I really liked it, even though I was never very good. No matter how hard I tried, I could never get my score down to an acceptable number. Being outdoors, enjoying the scenery and the people made it worthwhile and enjoyable.

Even though Antonio was generous on birthdays and holidays, I soon learned he was overly frugal on things he thought were frivolous or he didn't think were necessary. He limited giving me money toward general needs like haircuts, personal items, and clothes. He basically didn't give me much money for myself, which I found very frustrating since he always bought what he wanted. I decided I would look for a part-time job.

Castleton's, a family-owned business and upscale department store in the Olympus Hill shopping center was not far from our house. Antonio had a colleague from work whose wife was a buyer for them. She and I met at one of the company's outings, and she asked me to work there and model for them when needed. I usually worked afternoons or evenings and some Saturdays. I mostly worked in lingerie and women's departments, and I modeled clothes for the buyers, but mainly bras and lingerie. It was fun!

I soon learned I was pretty good at selling. Castleton's paid a salary plus commission, so I loved when the husbands came in, usually at the last minute, to buy gifts for their wives. I could talk most of them into buying anything. So, I sent them off with clothes, lingerie, perfume, and jewelry, all wrapped beautifully. The husbands were elated to take home such nice things.

However, it was not uncommon for some of the wives to come back the next week to exchange them. Most expressed their husbands had spent too much money, purchased things that didn't fit, or they didn't like.

Since I was still having female problems, I had to go in for some surgery on my bladder while living at the Olympus Hills house. The doctor performed a urethrotomy; the procedure requires them to cut a stricture of the urethra. The surgery made such a difference, and my urinary tract infections were less.

We wanted to have more children, but I hadn't been able to get pregnant yet. I was hoping this surgery would help me feel better.

One day, Antonio came home with a new motorcycle, a Yamaha dirt bike. He hadn't even discussed the idea with me, and I was shocked and hurt. He seemed to find the money for anything he wanted but still wouldn't even give me money for the basics. His logic was that he could save on gas and drive it to work when the weather was good. The idea of him driving in Salt Lake traffic didn't sit well with me. I was always afraid of people getting hit on motorcycles, but it didn't seem to bother him. So, life went on, and I continued to work at the department store, so I could still have my own spending money.

We lived in that house for about four years. We had nice neighbors and had a good time golfing in the warm months and skiing in the winter.

Antonio thought preschool was a waste of time and money, so I worked with Adrienne to get her ready for kindergarten.

She started school while we were living in Olympus Hills. She had friends in the neighborhood, so when school started, she was excited, and I cried. I was a typical mother, not wanting to see my little girl grow up. Antonio gave me some money to buy school clothes, but not as much as I felt was necessary. I sewed most of her clothes but also purchased some things for her from the money I earned at the store.

Money was always an issue between Antonio and me.

Antonio wanted to buy a duplex for an investment. He looked around for several months until he found one in the nearby city of Midvale that was only about a year old. The couple who owned it were getting a divorce, and it was not far from his parents' house. It was brick, well built, and had an unfinished basement that had plenty of space to add more rooms.

Everything was tastefully done, and we decided to sell our house and move into the duplex. We would rent out the other side to help with the mortgage.

We sold our house for about $25,000. Our profit was $4,000—we thought we had hit the mother lode! We were so elated to be able to move into the duplex.

Chapter Twelve

Life is not what you expect. It is made up of the most unexpected twists and turns.

—ILAIYARAAJA

One afternoon, I got a terrible pain that doubled me over. It was about the time we were trying to sell our house and close on the duplex. I didn't know what was happening. I felt different than I ever had before, so I called the doctor, and he told me to meet him at the hospital.

Antonio was at work, Adrienne was at school, so I went over to a neighbor's house for help. She offered to get Adrienne for me. When I reached Antonio by phone, he immediately left work to pick me up.

By the time we arrived at the hospital, I could hardly bear the pain. My doctor did some tests and soon determined I was having an ectopic pregnancy and would have to go into surgery. I had no idea I was even pregnant. My left fallopian tube had burst, and I was bleeding internally. They removed the left tube, ovary, and my appendix. I appreciated my doctor so much; when I awoke from surgery, he told me I was lucky I got in when I did as I could have bled to death. After spending several days in the hospital, I went home to recuperate.

We had been married five years, and I still hadn't conceived. Now my chances were less with only one tube and ovary left. I was sad. I came from a family of nine children. I loved babies, and I wanted to have more children. The whole experience caused me to go into depression. I would cry watching diaper commercials, or when I saw parents pushing their babies in strollers.

I quit my job with Castleton's since we were moving and would be too far away. We moved into the duplex, and I tried to put my energies into decorating our new house. The duplex was in a good location, not far from Antonio's work, close to his parents, and schools for Adrienne. I liked our new place and thought of ways we could eventually finish the basement. I think having a purpose helped me feel better, along with medication, of course.

A close friend from school in Pocatello decided to move next door in the other side of the duplex. She and her husband moved to Utah, so Kirk could go to law school. I was elated to have someone near me who I could confide in and do things with. My mood finally improved.

With Adrienne in school, I decided to look for another job. Before I was married, I had worked for a car dealership in Pocatello. Park Larsen Auto was not far from us in Midvale, so I applied for a part-time receptionist job. Greeting people and answering phones kept me busy, and the days went by fast.

Most days, I was home when Adrienne got home from school. I went about my domestic duties, worked, and tried not to think about having more children. I moved on, but there was always an ache in my heart.

Between working, being a mom and wife, I became interested in esoteric subjects. I read books on astrology, numerology, card reading, especially Tarot, and palmistry. They were fascinating, so I took classes to learn more. It all seemed so natural and easy to me, and I was amazed how accurate the information was. I joined an Astrology Association and started doing charts on family and friends. Word spread, and I found myself doing charts for anyone who was interested.

We didn't have computers, so everything was done manually. Esoteric books and newsletters helped me figure out how to do the charts. The charts were complicated, and it was important to have the correct information before I started one. I typed everything up, so I could give each person a copy; it also kept my typing skills sharp in case I needed them for another job.

I think some of my family thought I had lost my mind. Even though I was Catholic and many of the esoteric subjects are frowned upon, I soon learned they were a way of expanding our spiritual knowledge, not substituting any of it. I learned so much about myself and others, and found it an interesting, amazing outlet. I had always been intuitive, and everything I was learning helped me develop that intuition even more.

Chapter Thirteen

Life is full of surprises. You don't know what will happen, so enjoy and be ready for the surprises.
—AUTHOR UNKNOWN

When I got my interest in esoteric subjects, I started taking more classes. One class on Birth Control became of great concern for me since I hadn't been able to have more children. I figured I had nothing to lose, so I would try this new method of plotting when the best time was to conceive. I had it pinned down to when I could conceive and what sex it would be. When I got pregnant, I was as surprised as anyone else. Antonio looked at me in a different light and never questioned my *knowing* much after that.

We were elated. I was pregnant!

In 1973, tests were not done to determine the sex of the baby, except for high-risk patients. We had to wait nine months to find out whether we would have a boy or a girl. My doctor and I laughed when he bet me a six pack of beer that I would have a girl, and I said I was having a boy.

About the time we found out about the pregnancy, Antonio started experiencing odd symptoms. He was thirty years old, and we had been married about six years. His symptoms started with numbness in his hands and arms. He was a draftsman, so numbness was a big deal. He used his hands every day to draw plans for work, and now it was becoming difficult.

We were so excited about the new baby to come; we didn't think so much about his problem. He was in the prime of his life and couldn't imagine anything serious, so we assumed it was just a pinched nerve.

The doctor sent him for physical therapy a few days a week. He added massage, hot therapy treatments, and exercise, but none of it seemed to help. His symptoms compounded, he began having trouble walking, even stumbling like he was drunk even though he had never had a drink. Soon after, he started slurring his words and vision problems.

After one of his appointments with the eye doctor, Antonio went to see a neurologist. We both thought that was a little weird, but the eye doctor obviously could see things we couldn't and didn't want to scare us. He simply said additional tests would be more helpful.

We went through several months of tests, ruling out what Antonio didn't have, but there were not as many sophisticated machines and tests as there are today; Antonio just got worse. The not knowing was discouraging and frustrating.

Todd Antonio Amante was born on November 3, 1973, a beautiful boy, with a good set of lungs, and we couldn't have been happier.

I won the bet, and my doctor brought me a six pack of beer. We all laughed and forgot about Antonio's problem for a short period of time. Little Todd was healthy, and we were so grateful that God had blessed us with another child.

For a few months after Todd's birth, we enjoyed our *bundle of joy*. Such a happy baby, seldom crying, and woke up cooing to the delight of everyone in the family. Antonio's parents were so glad to have their first grandson that could carry on the Amante name.

Adrienne was elated to have a brother and was a big help. She could hardly wait to get home from school each day to play with him. They were eight years apart, and she loved him so much.

Right after the Thanksgiving and Christmas holidays that year, Antonio's doctor ordered a spinal tap. He was scheduled early in the day for the test, and back then, a patient had to lay on their stomach and not move their head for twenty-four hours. We waited for hours after Antonio's test, but the doctor never came in to talk to us, adding to our frustration of not knowing.

I was nursing Todd, and my breasts were so uncomfortable that if I didn't get home soon, I thought they would surely burst.

I finally left the hospital to go home, nurse baby Todd, and check on everything there. Antonio's parents were watching Adrienne and Todd, and they were as anxious to get the results as we were. The doctor left a message that he would talk to us in the morning, so I got to the hospital early, hoping to talk to the doctor and take Antonio home.

The doctor finally came in and broke the devastating news that Antonio's diagnosis was multiple sclerosis (MS).

We were in shock.

We didn't know much about the disease or what it could do to him. The doctor sent us home with a health plan and made an appointment for Antonio to see him again in a month.

We couldn't believe this was happening to us.

I soon started investigating every bit of information I could find about MS. I read books, articles, newsletters, health magazines, anything that might help us understand this disease. There was no cure for MS, so we had to figure out how to live with it knowing it would affect our entire family and change everything in our future.

The next year, we did anything and everything to make Antonio stronger. Physical therapy, exercises, vitamins, eating healthy, even juicing, and resting. It was a slow process.

At first, Antonio got worse, and it was very discouraging. His hands and legs were constantly tingling. He had to use a cane for balance. His eyesight got worse, and he started having exacerbations frequently which were extremely painful. Exacerbations are like an epilepsy attack; they only last for a minute, but they paralyzed him on one side while they lasted. He was given some medicine to help with those.

There were not as many medicines and treatments back then as there are today. The doctor did put him on a medication that did help with the exacerbations.

We tried nearly everything that we found to try to help with this ugly, crippling disease. We wanted so much for his life and ours to be back to normal. I became very protective of him and made sure he rested when tired, took his medicines, and was eating healthy.

Eventually, Antonio went into remission and remained there for nearly twenty years.

He never lost certain symptoms, fatigue, tingling in hands, arms, legs, but was able to keep the pain under control and learned to live with them. He had good days and bad days. If he was too tired, he rested. If he wasn't feeling well, he took it easy. Slowly, he became stronger and able to live some semblance of normal. He was able to go back to work full-time, to provide for his family, and made a big difference to him. To all of us.

Our prayers were answered when he felt good enough to snow ski, water ski, and golf again. He couldn't perform his favorite sports like he could before, but he could do them. This made him happy, hopeful, and determined to do all he needed to remain stable and healthy. He never complained and wasn't about to give in to weakness.

He didn't want to go to MS outings. He didn't want to see what the future might do to him. He was supportive but wanted to find his own path back to normalcy and life itself.

Life became somewhat normal again. We enjoyed our children and getting together with our family.

In the summer, we would golf, go camping or boating with his family, and take trips when possible. In the winter, we would ski or go snowmobiling. Most of the time was spent with his parents, brothers, or other extended family.

We would go to Idaho to see my family on occasion, especially at Thanksgiving. That was one time of year most of my siblings could get together at my mom's house. My mom made the best turkey, gravy, and stuffing, and we all looked forward to the meal. We would all make a special dish and eat until we were so full, we could hardly move. It was heaven, and a tradition carried on many years.

Many years, Antonio's parents and his Nonna would go with us. Everyone got along, and it was fun to look forward to that holiday. We would have a great time visiting and catching up on each other's lives.

One Thanksgiving when we went to Idaho, I was not feeling very well, and I didn't know what was going on. By the time we got back home, I hadn't improved and made an appointment with my doctor. After a few tests, the doctor confirmed I was having another ectopic pregnancy; only this time it was in my only ovary.

Typically, the egg cell is not released or picked up at ovulation but fertilized within the ovary where the pregnancy implants. This usually happens within the first four weeks of pregnancy.

Once again, I didn't know I was pregnant, so back to surgery to have it removed. The doctor did his best to repair the ovary, but my chances of getting pregnant again were slim. I was so sad, but I was grateful we had Adrienne and Todd.

Life went on.

Chapter Fourteen

Look deep into nature and then you will
understand everything better.

—ALBERT EINSTEIN

After Antonio was feeling stronger again, he decided we should buy a truck and camper, so we could enjoy more of the outdoors and get away more on summer weekends. We shopped dealerships for a few weeks and decided on a brand new 1973 GMC truck. It was green, and we found a camper that was green and white that looked great with the truck. This allowed us to spend more time with his family and friends and enjoy nature.

We loved southern Utah, so we took trips to Bryce Canyon, Zions, Moab, Canyonlands, and other national parks. We would often meet his extended family, especially at Redfish Lake, Mirror Lake, American Fork Canyon, or other beautiful spots near the mountains and lakes of Utah and Idaho.

We would spend hours by the campfire, cooking polenta, gnocchi, spaghetti, campfire dinners, roasting hot dogs, and making smores. Everyone looked forward to Grandpa Amanté's breakfasts with an abundance of fried potatoes, eggs, sausage, bacon, or ham. Lots of coffee topped off the menu. After eating, many of the family would go fishing, riding motor bikes, hiking, or stay in the campsite and read or visit.

We had good times, and I didn't mind it even though it was a lot of work to prepare the food and camper before going, and then cleaning everything up after returning home. It was worth it because the camper made it more comfortable and gave us some privacy when needed.

Antonio's Aunt Rena owned a flower shop, so I borrowed a long flower box from her. It made a perfect bed for the baby. The table could be made into a bed for Adrienne, and she slept there when she wasn't off with her cousins.

We have wonderful memories from those years, and our kids learned to love the outdoors and the wonders of nature.

Antonio and I had waited so long to have more children, and I just wanted to be home to raise Todd and Adrienne, so I quit my job at the dealership. Being home made it easier for me to take care of

Antonio. I did end up working part time for three different insurance agents all near our complex, and they allowed me plenty of flexibility. It worked out great and provided us with a little extra money.

In June 1975, Antonio and I played in a golf tournament in Wendover, Nevada. It was nice to be away from the kids for a few days, and we had a good time with friends. We enjoyed being together, just the two of us. We played golf, gambled, and had a nice dinner.

Soon after this trip, my breasts felt sore, and my body felt different. Could I be pregnant? I made an appointment with my doctor and confirmed I really was pregnant! We were both shocked! We didn't think we would ever have any more children; it was wonderful news to all of us.

Our third child, Robert Giovanni Amante was born on March 14, 1976. We were so excited to have another boy; he came out crying and never stopped. We knew miracles could happen, and we felt our family was complete.

Todd and Robert became the best of friends. They got along well and always played together; seldom ever fighting. Adrienne loved being a big sister and could hardly wait to get home from school to play with them. Since she was older, she was a big help to me. Those years were some of the happiest of my life.

As the kids grew up, we found ourselves running to soccer, basketball games, and golf tournaments. Antonio taught each of them to ski when they were about five. He had clubs cut down to fit them, so he could teach them to golf. They enjoyed these sports into their adult lives often spending time with us on the weekends. I believe those weekends contributed to our being a close family.

Chapter Fifteen

Families are the compass that guides us.
They are the inspiration to reach great heights and
our comfort when we occasionally falter.

—BRAD HENRY

In the late 1970's, Antonio was asked by his company if he would go to Pocatello for some contract work with Food Machinery Corporation (FMC). Since it was a big job and would last about a year, we decided to move to Pocatello. It meant I could spend more time with my family. Adrienne was in middle school, but the boys hadn't started school yet.

We decided to rent out the duplex and bought a house in Pocatello. My sister Sage, who was an engineer for the railroad, was making good money and agreed to buy it when the project was over. It was a perfect plan.

It was nice to spend more time with my family. We were able to see each other more often and to celebrate birthdays and holidays together. Adrienne played basketball in middle school, and our house was just across the street, so we went to most of the games as did many of my family. We all enjoyed watching her play.

When the project was over, we decided to keep the duplex as a rental and buy a house in Salt Lake. The house we liked was in Sandy, Utah, and was just being built. Most of it was done, but we were able to choose our own colors, carpet, appliances, counter tops, etc.

We lived in this house for over twenty-two years. Adrienne started high school at Alta High, and the boys at Sunrise Elementary which was practically in our backyard.

The school district had a good reputation, and it was in a new subdivision. We bought one of the first homes, so we had an opportunity to meet the new people as they moved in. Over the years, we had some wonderful neighbors, and our kids had plenty of friends.

Joanne and Cliff moved in next door, and to this day, they remain some of our best friends. They had two children, Calli and Zach.

Antonio's health was doing okay, so when he wasn't at his job, he worked on the house or yard. We put in a big garden, and over the years, finished landscaping the yard and finished the basement. We had plenty of room for our family.

All three of our kids graduated from Alta High. Adrienne had taken up track, and the boys did soccer, basketball, and golf.

Now that the kids were in school and Antonio's health was stable, I decided to look for a job. I was hired at Dale Carnegie Institute where I sold education classes. It was a great opportunity as I was able to take all their classes as well. I gained a lot of knowledge and confidence learning the Dale Carnegie philosophy.

There were three or four classes a year, so we agents would hustle to fill them. We were paid base plus commission. Sometimes it was a little sparse in between classes but gave us time to network and plan for the next class. It was fun working there, and I got to meet a lot of nice people in many different walks of life.

When Adrienne graduated from high school in 1983, I wanted to buy her a car, so she could get around when she found a job. Antonio was against it.

We argued so much over this issue, and the tension in the house led me to file for a divorce. I had had it with his frugal ways. He always got what he wanted but seldom did I get what I wanted. I was putting my foot down this time. I had always wanted to get Adrienne into dancing lessons, but he wouldn't let me. He didn't think preschool was necessary for Adrienne or the boys. There was always something he didn't think was necessary.

I think Antonio was shocked when I did go to an attorney. I filed for a separation, and he moved in with his parents. The kids were with me during the week, and he would take them on weekends. We were separated for about eight months, and the divorce was getting close to being final. Adrienne got a cute yellow Volkswagen Bug for her graduation present. She found a job that summer checking at Grand Central.

Then came Christmas with all the feelings, traditions, and sentiments of the holidays. The family memories, being together, all the love and fun of the past made my heart ache. I felt lost, abandoned, and hurt. Was this divorce really what I wanted?

On Christmas Eve, Antonio took the kids to his parents, and I was alone for the first time in my life on Christmas Eve. When Antonio and the kids came home, I was sitting by the fireplace drinking a glass (or two) of wine.

I could see in their eyes that they were sad I hadn't gone with them. The kids went to bed, and Antonio and I talked for a long time. We both realized how lonely we were, how much we missed each other. We decided to stop the divorce and get back together.

We went to his parents for Christmas day, and all the family were so glad we were together. It was a little awkward at first, but it didn't take long to feel normal again. That Christmas Day was a joyous and happy time for us, and we realized how much time we had wasted. We both knew how important communication was, and how important it was for us to be considerate of the other's desires and needs.

We spent New Year's Eve in Wendover, Nevada, with Antonio's brother Luca and his wife Jo. We had the best time. We got drunk, had a ton of fun, and by midnight, we were popping balloons and giving kisses. Luca and Jo bought a condo in Mesquite, so we added gambling and golf to the fun. This became our New Year holiday tradition.

Chapter Sixteen

Life presents many choices.
The choices we make determine our future.
—CATHERINE PULSIFER

My health issues never completely went away. I still had some concerns, and I was tired of pain and female problems, so I finally had a hysterectomy. The doctor tried to talk me out of it just in case something happened to Antonio. I might decide to remarry and want more children. I knew the chances were slim, and anyway, I just wanted to be done. After surgery, I felt much better. Looking back now, I think I had endometriosis, which wasn't diagnosed at that time.

Antonio was still able to work and do most things, but he had suffered frustrating issues with his MS over the years. He was often tired and needed to rest. He had bowel issues that prevented him from going places at times. MS affects almost everything in the body at certain times. But he was always hopeful and tried to be healthy and exercise, and he rarely complained.

In 1984, my sister Sage had a baby. She needed a nanny and hired Adrienne. It was a perfect arrangement; she could go to school at Idaho State University in Pocatello. Adrienne spent that year in school, lived with Sage, and took care of Tukker James.

I'm not too sure how Adrienne was feeling about school, as her grades weren't the best, but she did finish that first year there. Antonio and I had made a deal with her about grades. She would pay for the first semester, and we would reimburse 100% for A's, 75% for B's, 50% for C's. I'm not sure what the final tally was, but not as good as we had hoped.

Adrienne went back to school in Salt Lake choosing to major in the medical field. She continued her education at Westminster College in Salt Lake. She graduated on May 30, 1992, from nursing school and went on to intern in Montezuma, Utah. She achieved her Nurse Practitioner degree in May 1997, worked at Holy Cross Hospital in Salt Lake City for several years in labor and delivery, then a private female clinic of OB/GYN at the Avenues Women's Group. She went to the Huntsman Cancer Institute in the breast cancer division where she remains today. She was always concerned about her dad's health, and even with her busy schedule, she was always there to help when needed.

Chapter Seventeen

Risk something or forever sit with your dreams.
—HERB BROOKS

I decided I wanted to work for a company that had good benefits, and after investigating several occupations, I decided on a job at the airlines; good salaries, great benefits, and a chance to travel the world. I wanted to stay based in Salt Lake and was hired by Continental Airlines. The classes started in 1986 on November 3, Todd's birthday. I considered that a good omen. It was my goal to put part of my salary in a special fund for traveling, a main incentive with the airlines. We went to Las Vegas, many cities in Mexico such as Acapulco, Puerta Vallarta, Mazatlan, Zihuatanejo, Ixtapa, Cancun, Cozumel. In Hawaii, we visited Oahu, Maui, Kauai, and the Big Island. Those were the days when we could get on a plane as a non-rev. We were so fortunate Antonio's health was good enough for these trips, and we usually traveled first class.

A couple of years later, Continental decided to close their Salt Lake office. I had a chance to transfer to Houston, Texas, or one of their other hubs, but because of Antonio's health problems, we decided that wasn't a good idea. I needed to be close to home. I could be a flight attendant, but for the same reasons, I turned that down. So, I took the furlough, being confident that some other opportunity would come along, I watched for any job openings in other airlines. Delta was hiring, and I started on March 14, Robert's birthday. Again, a good omen. Working for the airlines was a blessing, and Antonio was happy I could contribute so much for the family.

I was with Delta for fourteen years before retiring, and some of my good friends from there I still see today.

I started as a reservation agent, and my work for Continental made it much easier for me to transition to a different company. Over the years, I worked as a trainer, went on the International reservations desk, and worked at the Skymile desk. Even though it was challenging at times, I loved my job. Between Continental and Delta, I made good money, had great health benefits, plus travel, making the difficulty of Antonio's disease a little easier to bear. It was a great job, and I was very grateful to have it.

Adrienne and Aaron were married on September 5, 1992, in the quaint chapel at Holy Cross Hospital where Adrienne was working at the time. They had a lovely reception at the Millcreek Inn. Aaron was amazing and fit right into our family; he could fix anything. They bought a house in Sugarhouse, so we saw them often. Antonio really liked Aaron, and they bonded together just like any father and son relationship.

Antonio had always wanted to go to Italy where most of his ancestors were born. His health was starting to deteriorate as he was having a hard time walking. Adrienne was working, so she couldn't go with us, but Todd and Robert came. We borrowed an old wheelchair of his dad's, hoping we could get Antonio around easier. Little did we realize that pushing a wheelchair on cobblestone streets was not easy. Antonio didn't like being in the wheelchair but knew it was the only way for him to get around.

We flew into Milan, Italy, and took a train to Lugano, Switzerland. Someone at work had told me it was a charming city and worth a visit; he was right. Our hotel was only a few blocks from the train station. Across the street from the hotel was an Italian restaurant where we went for dinner that night. The food was so delicious. Antonio had lasagna, and the chef made the best mushroom gnocchi I had ever tasted.

It was a fun city, and the next day, we all enjoyed our walk around beautiful Lake Lugano.

Chapter Eighteen

Traveling—it leaves you speechless,
then turns you into a storyteller.

—IBN BATTUTA

Rome is a fascinating city as it is so old and has so many interesting places to see. We had a private tour guide named Gabriella. She was a young French girl who spoke very good English. For three days, we would meet her at the bus stop which was just around the corner from our hotel. Each day, we would go to a different area to see the sights of the city. We saw beautiful churches, the Vatican, the Catacombs, the Colosseum, the Roman Forum, the fountains, and the Pantheon. Antonio couldn't go into the Catacombs as it is underground and has very narrow pathways. Gabriella brought a book and sat with Antonio explaining it to him and showing pictures. The boys and I went inside. The Catacombs is an underground ancient burial cemetery. I didn't like it much. I found it creepy and felt the spirits of the deceased.

So many bodies were buried in small spaces. Burials had to be done that way as there were so many people and so little space. It is so different from the burials of today.

The Colosseum looked like a crumbling bunch of ruins, but the history there was fascinating. It was built in 80 AD, right in the center of the city.

"Antonio, can you believe entertainment consisted of men fighting each other or beasts like lions and tigers?"

Antonio said, "I heard the Colosseum held 60,000 people and had around 450 years of service. The higher areas were ruined by fires and earthquakes. When the Roman empire began to falter, and games were too expensive to hold, by the tenth century, the Colosseum had been abandoned. Tourists by the thousands come every year to look at the history of ancient Rome."

"Wow, it's hard to believe anything could last that long," said Todd.

We saw many other sites such as the Roman Forum, the famous fountains of Rome, like Trevi Fountain, the Pantheon, and the Vatican. Being Catholic, the Vatican and Saint Peter's Basilica were of special interest to us.

I felt so spiritual there and wanted all my sins forgiven and felt the need to be an even better Catholic. At least, temporarily until I arrived back home where I lost some of that desire.

Antonio was excited to see all the sights he had studied over the years. The boys had taken art history and found it fascinating to see pictures and sculptures they had studied in school.

Saint Peter's Basilica is breathtaking, and the Sistine Chapel puts us in awe of the talent that went into all of it. The beauty and stories brought tears to my eyes. Antonio and the boys were just as in awe as I was.

The Papel Audience is held weekly, and the Pope rides around in his *Pope Mobile,* and delivers his weekly message to the people attending. The Pope at the time was Pope Paul II. He reigned as Pope of the Roman Catholic Church and sovereign of the Vatican City for nearly 27 years (1978-2005).

It was a very hot day, and we were in line for hours before the ceremony started. I was worried about Antonio and whether he could physically hold up. Finally, the time arrived, and the Pope came by us. We were right in front of the line where the car passed by. The Pope stopped right in front of us and blessed Antonio. I got a beautiful picture. It was so emotional for all of us to be that close to the Holy

Man. Antonio had tears in his eyes, and I was overcome with spirituality and awe. It was an amazing experience to be there to see and hear the Pope so close to us. Even our boys were touched.

As we were leaving the Vatican, we saw many people who had made a pilgrimage there. One kind soul came up to Antonio, blessed him, and gave him a holy medal. It was quite an experience for all of us, and one we will never forget.

Inside, we went to the Sistine Chapel. The Sistine ceiling and the Last Judgment by Michelangelo decorate the interior. So much is going on in the picture that you could spend hours studying it. It is amazing to see, just breathtaking.

Antonio said, "This is one of the sights I particularly wanted to see. It is so beautiful," and Robert agreed.

Between 1508 and 1512, Michelangelo painted the Chapel's ceiling, a project that changed the course of Western Art. It is regarded as one of the major accomplishments of human civilizations. Thousands of tourists come to see the beautiful work every year.

Antonio, Todd, Robert, and I were so glad to share this experience.

While we were in Rome, we found some wonderful Italian food and had our first taste of gelato. It was so delicious that we went every day to get one.

At that time, gelato was not as well known in the states as it is now. It was the first time we had tasted it, and from then on, it became a favorite dessert. It is so delicious, a lot like ice cream, but creamier and has more fruit. All of us became obsessed with having gelato every day.

Our visit to Rome was very fulfilling, exciting, and wonderful to see so many interesting places for our first trip to Europe. We were so grateful we were able to be there.

Chapter Nineteen

I believe that whether a person
follows any religion or not is unimportant—
he/she must have a good heart, a warm heart.

—DALAI LAMA

By the time we got on the plane, we were all exhausted, but a good kind of tired. Antonio was elated and fell asleep right away.

I couldn't sleep on the plane. I never could sleep on an airplane. Antonio was sleeping next to me, and the boys were in the row in front of us. Robert had his light on and was reading. He came back to me, and I could see he was shaking.

"What is the matter?" I asked.

He said, "The weirdest thing happened to me while I was reading. I'll be right back."

He went to the bathroom and was there for several minutes. I was getting concerned, but he finally came back. He said, "Mom, I had to go into the bathroom to pray. I got down on my knees and prayed to God. I felt the Holy Spirit."

Not knowing quite what to say at that time, I said to him, "We will talk more about this when we get home."

In my heart, I was hoping he felt the spirituality of being at the Vatican, seeing the Pope, and inviting us in our Catholic religion. I was in for a big surprise when we got home.

Chapter Twenty

> *You cannot change the circumstances, the seasons,*
> *or the wind, but you can change yourself. That is*
> *something you are in charge of. Life is an unending*
> *stream of extenuating circumstances.*
>
> —AUTHOR UNKNOWN

A few days after we got back from Europe, Robert came over to talk to me about his experience on the plane. He just wanted to talk to me and not his dad at that time. He wasn't sure how his dad would take it and didn't want to upset him. He told me he had been reading *The Book of Mormon* on the plane. He had many Mormon friends over the years, and I never thought much about it since they were good guys, and they all had fun together both in school and out.

Robert was presently living at the Sigma Chi fraternity house while in his senior year at the University of Utah. He was majoring in Finance and

Business and had gotten nearly a 4.0 grade point average all throughout his college days. He was smart, like his dad.

Robert told me again how he had felt the Holy Spirit when he was on the plane and had gone to the bathroom to pray. He said that his fraternity brothers had been talking a lot about God and questioning their existence on earth. They had several nights where they discussed the subjects. One of his Mormon friends told him he should read the *Book of Mormon.*

Robert told me he wanted to talk to the missionaries to understand the Mormon religion better. Robert asked me not to say anything to Dad yet as he wasn't sure how he would take it.

I told him it was fine to explore spirituality and other religions, but not to make any rash decisions. I felt it was interesting to study other religions and cultures to see how they varied from our own Catholic religion. We can never get too much knowledge.

A few weeks later, Robert came over again and told me he wanted to be baptized in the Mormon religion. At first, I was hurt, having raised him in the Catholic religion and felt we must have failed him in some way. I told him if he was doing it for the right reason that I could learn to accept his decision. I didn't want him to be baptized so he could be with a Mormon girl, but because he believed in why he was making this change. We waited until he had planned with the church before we told Antonio.

Robert was ready to tell his dad about his decision and the rest of the family. Antonio was the least surprised of any of the family and told Robert to follow his heart, he took the news better than anyone, much to our surprise.

When the rest of the family was told about the decision, they were not happy. They couldn't understand why he would want to change from the Catholic religion he was brought up in. Antonio told us Robert was an adult and could make his own decisions to follow his dream.

I told Robert if that was the decision he chose, I could live with it because I loved him too much and would never want to lose him. But we had conditions; Robert was not to come home and preach to us or try to convert us to his new religion. If the family was drinking wine, alcoholic drinks, or other things the Mormons didn't believe in, he must accept that as being part of the family.

None of us felt comfortable going to his baptism, but we all wished him well. I was hurt for a long time, but because Robert kept up his end, we were able to continue as a family, and it worked out.

Knowing that Antonio accepted Robert's decision made it easier for the kids and me.

Chapter Twenty-One

Things change. Stuff happens. Life goes on.

—Author Unknown

Not long after we got back from Europe, Antonio became weaker and was having more trouble walking. He had been sleeping downstairs, and I was upstairs. One day, he fell out of bed and broke his hip.

I could hear him hollering, so I ran downstairs, and there he was on the floor. I immediately called 911 when I realized he was hurt and couldn't move.

He was operated on but afterward was paralyzed from the neck down. He went to rehab for several weeks, and then we were able to take him home.

He could move his head, but he had no feeling nor couldn't move his arms, legs, or body.

It was heartbreaking. His mind was still sharp, so he was aware of everything that was happening to him and around him. All these years he had MS, neither of us ever imagined this.

He would be bed bound and totally dependent on others to take care of his every need. Shower him, shave him, brush his teeth and hair, dress him, and feed him. Every personal thing we do for ourselves, Antonio now had to have it done for him, not assisted, done for him.

We took care of his every need each day to make his life comfortable and to show him we loved him.

One of Antonio's greatest concerns was taking care of our family. Even though Adrienne was married, and Todd and Robert were living away from home, he still wanted to make sure we were all cared for. But Antonio was smart, frugal, and we had planned for our future. We had rental properties, good investments, and a diversified portfolio that we had worked on our whole married life. We had good insurance through Delta Air Lines, and he would qualify for disability, while I would continue working.

Now that our income had changed, and Antonio would not be able to take care of the house anymore, we decided to sell. We found a nice condo in the Holladay area and had it completely remodeled to be wheelchair accessible. It took a few months to complete, but we were excited to move to a smaller place.

Antonio was trying to adjust to his new circumstances as we all were. He accepted the fact that he would always need help for everything. Our family tried to obtain what was necessary to care for him. We purchased several items to help make our lives easier. A wheelchair, shower chair, and eventually we bought a van with a lift for the wheelchair when traveling to the doctor or other places. It made getting around so much easier.

The van purchase was made after several accidents when Antonio ended up on the ground. Before the van, when I took him to the doctor, there were times when attempting to get him from the car to the wheelchair, he slipped off the board and landed on the ground. I would have to find someone to help him.

A hospital bed soon became essential. We set one up in the second bedroom. Antonio was not happy about this arrangement, he wanted me next to him, but it was for his safety and the safety and ease for all who cared for him. We had to make it as easy as possible to get him in and out of bed. Antonio wanted me to sleep by him, but I had to convince him he had to be in a bed where it was easier to get him in and out.

I was still working for Delta Air Lines, so on days I worked, our kids would take turns coming over and spend the evening with their dad. They would feed him, get him ready for bed, and visit. These times became special and meaningful to all of us.

Antonio loved having Adrienne, Todd, and Robert come over on those days. The kids talked about life, movies, how school was going, or just everyday events. They watched TV or listened to music. Sometimes Robert would play the guitar for his dad.

Lots of memories were built, and they were all able to show their love. I bless these kids of ours for being there for us. I don't know if we would have been able to keep him at home without their help. It was hard work, and some days I would be so exhausted, but we all learned to do things we didn't know we could do. God helped us get through this difficult time, and I thank him every day for his help.

The priest from our church would come over once a week to visit us. Antonio enjoyed those visits. If there was anything to discuss about the future, it was nice to have the priest bring it up rather than me. The priest could talk about whether he was to be cremated or buried. He could ask questions that were hard for me. We were able to plan, and that was essential.

Antonio was in and out of the hospital several times usually for infections. He would no sooner get over one infection after taking antibiotics and another would come. The infections were difficult to cure because there were so many different kinds, but the worst was sepsis.

The doctor finally told us that there was nothing more he could do and recommended he be put on hospice. We kept him home, and they would come in and help. Hospice is a wonderful organization, and I have a lot of respect for the work they do, I'm not sure how I would have made it otherwise.

They showed me how to care for him, how to change his catheter, and redress any wounds he had, mostly bedsores. The first few times I changed his catheter, I had a hard time getting in, and blood squirted all over. I felt so bad and was grateful that he couldn't feel it. I showered him while the helpers would change his bed and get his required treatments ready. It worked out well.

Once he started losing his eyesight, television became difficult for him to watch. I would put on his favorite music and often read to him. We discussed books he might like, and I would read a little each day. He enjoyed that activity, and it kept him calm. He enjoyed biographies, and we read about the Kennedys. I would often get some inspirational stories that he enjoyed.

When it was warm and sunny outside, I would take him for a walk around the neighborhood. He often said fresh air and sun on his face felt so good to him. Some days I would put him in his wheelchair, and we would walk over to our dear friends Kathy and Paul who lived a few blocks away. It would pass the time for us both and helped alleviate boredom. Antonio seldom complained. He had a great attitude most days.

One day, Antonio woke up extremely grumpy and was being verbally mean to me. I was crushed. I looked into Antonio's eyes, with tears in mine, and said to him. "Antonio, you can't talk to me like that. Not only has your life changed but so has mine and all our family. I'm devastated that we will never be able to be the same again or do the things we used to do. I love you, and I will take care of you, but I can't take it if you are mean or grumpy. I'm doing the best I can."

I cried and was so hurt, but it must have gotten to him because he never did it again.

Chapter Twenty-Two

*Babies are like suns that, in a magical way, bring
warmth, happiness and light into our lives.*

—Kartini Diapari Ongider

Adrienne and Aaron had been trying to get pregnant but were not having much luck. They decided to try artificial insemination, but that didn't go well. Next, they did in vitro fertilization and even tried twice, but to no avail.

Adrienne was working at the time for an OB/GYN office. One day, a young teenager came in pregnant, and her parents didn't want her to keep the baby because she was so young. She didn't have long to go before her due date, so she had to make some difficult decisions.

It all happened so fast, but Adrienne and Aaron decided to adopt the baby. Aaron was working out of town and had to rush home to sign papers to get the process started. They didn't want to tell anyone but me, until they were sure the adoption would go through. It all went smoothly, and they got their baby girl, Jane on October 18, 1998.

I was at work, they called me, and I went to their house to see my first grandchild. I was so excited! Baby Jane was beautiful and warmed my heart completely. We felt so blessed to have her come into our lives at this time. Adrienne wanted to surprise Antonio and the rest of the family. So, we planned a get-together the next day at our condo.

It was all I could do to keep my mouth shut until the time came. We invited Todd and Robert, Antonio's parents and his brothers and their wives to come over for pizza.

When Antonio took his nap that day, I told him I had a surprise for him when he woke up. He thought I was making him a favorite dessert.

The boys came over first to meet their niece, Jane. They were so cute with her, and they were excited to be uncles. I got Antonio up and wheeled him into the family room. Adrienne and Aaron were standing with the baby in their arms.

Antonio looked up in amazement and asked, "Whose baby is that?"

Adrienne started to cry. "Hi, Grandpa, this is Jane, your first grandchild."

Antonio cried, too. "This gives me hope."

Hope is what we all needed at that time.

Adrienne helped her dad hold the baby since he didn't have use of his arms. It was so touching, and we were all in tears. Happy tears.

After about an hour of fighting over who got to hold Jane, we called the rest of the family over. Mom and Dad, Luca and Jo, Thomas, and Sue. When Mom and Dad walked in, they were very puzzled.

Bianca asked, "Whose baby is that? Are you babysitting someone's baby?"

Adrienne said, "Say hello to your first great-grand-daughter, Jane."

Bianca and Antonio Sr. thought they were teasing them. They were shocked, but when they realized it was real, they were so excited, and they cried, too.

Throughout the next year, baby Jane spent the day with us at least once a week while Adrienne and Aaron worked. I would tuck baby Jane into Antonio's arms in his bed, so he could cuddle her and talk to her. They often took naps together. It made Antonio so happy, and he looked so forward to the days when baby Jane could be with us. He would often ask me throughout the week if it was our day to have the baby. He couldn't wait to see her.

Chapter Twenty-Three

*Sometimes you have to accept
the fact that certain things will never go back
to how they used to be. Life goes on.*

—AUTHOR UNKNOWN

In November 1998, the whole family planned a trip to Maui, Hawaii, one of our favorite places. Antonio wanted to go one more time. Even though he was bedbound, we knew we could get him around with his wheelchair. We did not know at the time of the booking that we would have a new little baby with us that was only a few weeks old. After consulting doctors and the airlines, we were able to get the approval we needed for our entire family to go on the trip.

Antonio's mom and dad, his brothers and their wives, Thomas's two boys, Antonio, Todd, Robert, Adrienne, Aaron, baby Jane, and I packed up and headed for Hawaii. We enjoyed the sunshine and warm weather. We had a blast playing volleyball, going to the beach, and just having fun.

We got cabanas, so Antonio and Jane wouldn't be in the sun too much. We had been to Hawaii so many times over the years, so this time we just relaxed, no pressure to do much, and enjoyed being together.

In the mornings, I would sneak in Adrienne and Aaron's room and steal baby Jane. I would take her over to our room and cuddle her in bed next to Antonio. He loved it. Baby Jane was getting very spoiled quickly with so much attention. Everyone wanted to hold her and play with her. This trip was a very memorable one, and we got lots of pictures with baby Jane. Antonio loved being with all his family, and baby Jane brought him Joy. He was enjoying himself and the beautiful feel of Hawaii.

One of my favorite things to do in Hawaii is sit on the lanai in the morning, drink coffee, look out at the vast ocean, and listen to the waves. It is so peaceful. After getting Antonio ready for the day, I would wheel him out there to enjoy the fresh air and view. He couldn't see much by this time, but he saw shadows and enjoyed the fresh air and sound of the waves.

Before we left for the trip, I had worried if I could take care of him without the nurses. Fortunately, I had learned to change his catheter, redo his wounds, and bathe him. I had lots of help to move him around, and we all made it work. This trip was one of our most memorable ones, and we were so thankful we got to spend cherished time with Antonio. When it was time to go home, Antonio didn't want to leave. We all knew this would be his last trip to Hawaii. I thank God it was such a fun and meaningful trip for all of us.

In February 1999, Bianca died of an aneurysm. It happened so suddenly, leaving everyone in shock. We had a typical Catholic funeral, and Antonio was able to attend. He was devastated as he was always close to his mother. The funeral was hard on him and difficult for everyone to see how Antonio had deteriorated.

In my mind, I think Bianca wanted to die before her firstborn son. She was heartbroken when Antonio was first diagnosed with the disease and worried about him constantly.

It was a sad time.

After the funeral, Antonio began to deteriorate even further. The doctors said there were no further treatments to help. In May after a doctor's appointment, he was sent back home for hospice and his family to take care of him. He was given up to six months to live.

We both knew one day it would come to this. Even though he had multiple sclerosis most of his adult life, it was so painful to know he didn't have long to live. We all tried to make his life as comfortable as possible, but I was devastated to know we had reached this point.

Chapter Twenty-Four

We understand the miracle of life
when we allow the unexpected to change us.
—PAULO COELHO

Todd was taking the deterioration of his dad harder than anyone. It was hard on *everyone,* but I noticed it in him more. Todd was a man of few words, but he started questioning if God really existed. He couldn't understand why a loving God would allow his children to suffer like Antonio had. Everything he had been taught as a Catholic didn't seem to matter. Todd was angry and wasn't sure if he believed in God anymore. It hurt me to see Todd this way, and I didn't know how to comfort him.

Todd was always easygoing and quiet. He didn't like confrontations. He was always thinking and very smart, much like his dad. He graduated from the University of Utah in Mass Communications. After a few years of different jobs, and after his dad died, he decided to go back to school at the Golf Academy in San Diego. He studied to be a Golf Pro and went on to be a pro at various golf courses in Salt Lake City. They both loved the game of golf, and Todd knew his dad would be proud.

Our three children never hesitated to help their dad, especially once he was in hospice. They took care of his needs, talked with him about life, and spent valuable time with him. They were all a blessing to me as I was still working for Delta. We all created meaningful and comforting memories during those few months.

It wasn't long after Antonio was put on hospice that Robert came to me and said he wanted to go on a mission for his new religion, The Church of Jesus Christ of Latter-day Saints. I told him this was not the time as his dad was dying. He said he didn't think it would happen until after his dad was gone. Without us knowing, he turned in the request to go to an international destination. He thought it would take months to get approved, especially since he was a convert.

As life is always full of surprises, within a short period of time, he got called to do his mission in Sao Paulo, Brazil. In October, he was to report to the Missionary Training Center (MTC) in Provo, Utah, to learn Portuguese. I was not happy, and neither was the rest of the family once they knew of Robert's intentions. We just couldn't believe he could leave while his dad was dying. Robert was torn. He wanted to be here with his dad, but felt God was calling him to do his work.

Robert had a long talk with his dad, and Antonio told him, "Don't wait for me. You need to do what your heart tells you. You can make your own decisions now."

Everyone in the family was upset and couldn't believe he was really going to go, but Antonio gave Robert the courage to move forward.

The MTC was in Provo, Utah, so Robert wouldn't be too far away for several weeks. In October when he was done with his studies there, we gave him a farewell party. We knew he wouldn't be home for two years.

It was time to fly to Sao Paulo, Brazil. We were able to put Antonio in his wheelchair and take him to the airport to send Robert off. It was extremely emotional. Robert took his dad aside and had a talk with him, telling his dad he loved him, he would pray for him and would make him proud. They both cried, we all cried, and both Robert and Antonio knew it was their last time to be together in this life.

Chapter Twenty-Five

In one sense there is no death. The life of a soul on earth
lasts beyond departure. You will always feel that life
touching yours, that voice speaking to you. He lives on
in your life and in the lives of all others that knew him.

—ANGELO PATRI

As Antonio grew weaker, he started seeing and
hearing things from the spiritual world. Many
times, I would come into his room, he would ask me
if I had seen any of them.

"Is Nonna still here?" he would ask.

"No, I don't see her."

"Oh, there she is sitting in that chair," he said.

Nonna had been dead for several years.

Sometimes, Antonio would see his Nonno as well,
mostly always Nonna or Nonno. I would hear him
talking, and when I went in to check on him, it was
one of them he was talking to.

One morning around nine o'clock, I went into his

room to wake him up, which was our daily routine. Antonio asked if he could have a beer.

"Antonio, it is nine o'clock in the morning."

"I don't care. I just had one with your mom, and it tasted so refreshing, I'd like another one."

"Okay, beer instead of coffee this morning."

I didn't question him as I knew my mom loved her beer, and I could just picture them sitting together, chatting, and drinking a beer. Mom had died in 1991 from lung cancer.

I had no doubts that these people Antonio saw were real. He would describe in detail many of his visitors. It was chilling and yet comforting at the same time. Knowing others were around to meet him when the time came to go to the other side. It was reassuring to know they were there to help him. I was a believer.

In 1999, we had Thanksgiving at our condo. My sisters Lilly, Sage, and Lulu came from Idaho to spend it with us. We all knew this would be the last Thanksgiving with Antonio. My sisters and I drank a little too much wine at dinner to numb the reality and sadness, knowing Antonio would be gone soon. We tried to make the dinner lighthearted and fun.

While my sisters were there during the week, they would take turns bringing Antonio coffee in the morning and help him sip it while they chatted. He liked that a lot. He had always gotten along with my sisters. He enjoyed their good sense of humor and their perspective on life.

After they left, we went back to our daily routines. One thing we both liked was me reading to him. One of our favorite books was *Tuesdays with Morrie* by Mitch Albom. We were nearly done with the book and were looking forward to the movie coming out on television on December 5.

Even though Antonio had lost his eyesight, he could still hear. We would be done with the book before the movie was out.

Chapter Twenty-Six

*For life and death are one, even as
the river and the sea are one.*

—KAHLIL GIBRAN

On the morning of December 5, I woke Antonio at the usual time of 9 a.m. He seemed a little disoriented that morning and wasn't feeling good. I got him cleaned up, fed him his breakfast, and let him go back to sleep. When I went back to check on him, he was not responding to me. He had slipped into a coma. I called Adrienne, Aaron, and Todd to come over. When they arrived, he still was not responding. We called the rest of the family to come over.

As the day went on, nothing changed. Each person in the family went in alone and talked to him. They were all able to tell him their goodbyes, which was a blessing.

It had been a long day, and we were all tired. Around 7 p.m., I told everyone to go home, and if anything happened, I would call them. Adrienne and baby Jane were going to sleep over to be with me. After everyone left, I cleaned up the house while Adrienne put the baby to sleep in my bedroom. I was glad they were there as I was kind of numb and in shock. Even though we knew for months that Antonio would leave us, it still felt unbelievable it was time.

Just before 8 p.m., I went back into Antonio's room. I tried talking to him, but again, I got no response. I told him I was going to turn on the TV to watch the movie *Tuesdays with Morrie*.

About a half hour into the movie, Antonio started having labored breathing. As I listened to him up close, he took his last breath. I called Adrienne in to check him as well. We both agreed he was gone, so I called the hospice nurse to confirm that he was. Once the nurse announced he was dead, I called the rest of the family.

Was this really happening?

I had such a hollow feeling. Even though we knew for months that Antonio could go at any time, I was still shocked to think he was really gone. The sadness overwhelmed me, but I knew he was not suffering any more. All the pain and limited use of his body were finally over.

Antonio had gone through so much in his life-time, and the past two years were extremely difficult.

He didn't want to die, he loved his family, but he knew he had no choice. He was with God and his family who had gone before him.

Antonio was finally at peace.

Chapter Twenty-Seven

Accept what is, let go of what was,
and have faith in what will be.

—AUTHOR UNKNOWN

He had asked to be cremated, and we planned a traditional Catholic funeral. The priest who always came to visit him performed the ceremony. The funeral was held in the beautiful St. Ambrose Church in Sugarhouse. Planning the date of the funeral was a little awkward as Antonio died on December 5 and my birthday was on December 9. I didn't want my birthday to be the day of the funeral, so we decided on December 12. This allowed people from out of state to be able to attend.

In the process of planning the funeral, I called Robert's bishop and asked if he could come home for the funeral. Normally, once a missionary commits, they must stay there for two years. I told them how distraught we all were and how much we wanted

Robert there. I told them I worked for an airline, and I would get him home at our cost. If he could just come home for a week, I would make sure he went back. The bishop talked it over with some of the higher ups in the church and explained our feelings. Because he was a convert, they realized it was a different situation, and since Robert had not been assigned a companion yet, they allowed him to come home. One of the men of the Quorum of the Twelve called me. He couldn't have been nicer, more understanding, or helpful. I was so appreciative.

The whole family was so grateful, and we all felt so much relief knowing Robert would be there at the funeral. It was indeed a blessing after a difficult time.

The church-setting funeral was perfect, and we had chosen some beautiful music to play. "Ave Maria" and "Silent Night" were two of the songs we chose for a dear friend to sing.

Since it was close to the Christmas season, "Silent Night" seemed so appropriate. Every time I hear these songs, I think of Antonio and all the other family members who went before.

It was a very touching and emotional service.

Chapter Twenty-Eight

Enjoy life today, yesterday is gone and
tomorrow may never come.

—AUTHOR UNKNOWN

I now realize what is important. Life is a temporary state, and time goes by too quickly. We must learn to enjoy every precious moment. Celebrate life, birthdays, weddings, baptisms, holidays, or anything that is important to you and your family. Enjoy just being together with loved ones. We don't have time for all the hurts, misconceptions, and misunderstandings. We need to learn to take the high road and be the best person we can.

As I look back over the experience of living with someone who had multiple sclerosis, I learned many lessons about why they act like they do.

There are many ups and downs, and the disease of MS affects most everything in the body at different times, some at the same time, but everything is impacted. I believe one knowing how quickly life could change from good to worse, puts a heavy strain on the mind of those dealing with the disease. You must have faith and hope, and take care of yourself as best you can. You will have good times and bad times, but you learn to adjust to what is going on at that moment. You can live a fulfilling life and be happy despite the disease. Be positive!

Things in life change, and as a result, you change. You learn how to compensate for those changes. It is possible to be happy and feel blessed. Some days you almost forget that your loved one is sick, and things appear normal. You substitute one thing for another when necessary, but you never give up hope.

Somedays between work and taking care of him, I got so burned out I didn't know if I could do it anymore. Those were days I had to step back and do a mental adjustment, and you will, too.

Yes, I could tell you many stories, but that isn't important. I want to leave you with hope and know that you can make the most of each day, good or bad.

There were so many stolen moments in our life, but Antonio and I shared thirty-three years together despite the changes. After we were married, our life was filled with many of the things we enjoyed like skiing, golfing, boating, camping, and traveling. Antonio was in remission for many of those thirty-three years, and that allowed us to be encouraged and still do many of the things we wanted to do.

What could have been a promising future became a time of many stolen moments, but we still had a lot to look forward to and enjoy. We learned to appreciate every moment of every day despite the many adjustments. We did have a good life.

Just a few of those Stolen Moments . . .

Our life as we planned before the disease. We had planned to travel more and enjoy life.

We talked about opening an Italian restaurant or deli. We even thought of a bed and breakfast. All these choices took energy that we didn't have.

Sex and intimacy changed.

Physical activities were more limited, and we gave up many of those we enjoyed as a family.

Meaningful time we could have spent together besides going to doctors and hospitals.

Antonio, my beloved husband is gone...
The most difficult stolen moment!

I now know there is more to experience after this life. We have the afterlife to look forward to and be with our loved ones again. It is encouraging to know that we can be whole, without worries and pain and be healthy and happy once again.

God bless you dear souls.

Chapter Twenty-Nine

*The purpose of life is to live it, to taste experience
to the utmost, to reach out eagerly and without
fear for newer and richer experience.*

—AUTHOR UNKNOWN

20 THINGS THAT YOU CAN PRACTICE TO ENJOY MORE EVERY DAY:

1. Practice gratitude
2. Work on mindfulness
3. Put yourself first
4. Be kind to others
5. Celebrate small wins
6. Rest and recuperate
7. Invest in yourself
8. Nurture positive relationships
9. Meet new people
10. Consume less news and social media

11. Try new things

12. Get rid of clutter

13. Spend money on experiences, not possessions

14. Exercise regularly

15. Spend time in nature

16. Track your time

17. Cultivate a purpose

18. Contribute to others

19. Overcome destructive habits

20. Commit to mastering something

– AUTHOR UNKNOWN

ECCLESIASTES 3:1–8

To every thing there is a season, and a time to every purpose under the heaven.

A time to be born, and a time to die; a time to plant, and a time to pluck up that which is planted.

A time to kill, and a time to heal; a time to break down, and a time to build up.

A time to weep, and a time to laugh; a time to mourn, and a time to dance.

A time to cast away stones, and a time to gather stones together; a time to embrace and a time to refrain from embracing.

A time to get, and a time to lose; a time to keep, and a time to cast away.

A time to mend, and a time to sew; a time to keep silence, and a time to speak.

A time to love, and a time to hate; a time of war and a time of peace.

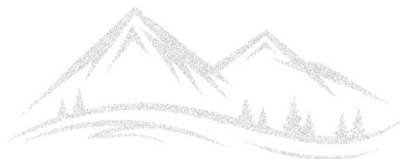

Epilogue

Twenty-three years have passed since Antonio left us. I never remarried; I dated but had a difficult time finding someone I wanted to be with forever. I couldn't see being with a man unless he could enhance my life, someone who I had a lot in common with and enjoyed doing the same things I wanted to do and accept my family.

Learning to be alone had its advantages and I found solitude rather inviting at times.

Thank God for my family and friends when I needed others around me.

My children, I'm a grandma now, and I enjoy all of them so much. Adrienne has three girls, Todd married and has two girls, and Robert married and has one girl and three boys. They are the sunshine in my life. I love them so much.

I've had a good life since Antonio died, but at times I have to admit I have been lonely. I miss having someone to talk to during meals and talk over problems that need to be solved. But I especially miss the intimacy, having someone to cuddle with and keep me warm in my bed.

After I retired from Delta Air Lines, I decided to build a log home. Antonio and I had bought property in beautiful Midway, Utah, about fifteen minutes from Park City. We were going to build, but then his illness got worse, so it never happened.

With the help of my sons and son-in-law doing some of the work along with the contractors, it took a couple of years to build. After it was finished, I moved in and lived there alone for ten years.

ACKNOWLEDGEMENTS

I want to thank Richard Paul Evans, my teacher and mentor. He gave me so much helpful information for writing my first book.

When I first met Richard at a book signing, I talked to him about wanting to write a book. I have been a fan of his since he wrote *The Christmas Box* and have read most of his books. I followed him on social media and when he started the Author Ready Group, I was one of the first to sign up. I was so excited to have access to many writing subjects at an affordable price.

After getting involved with the lessons, zoom meetings, and anything offered that I could attend, I got serious about writing my book. I went to my first writer's retreat in June 2022 at his Timepiece Ranch in southern Utah. I met so many wonderful people and I was impressed they were all so supportive to each other. My book started coming together with all their help.

Thank you to Richard, to Diane Glad, his assistant, who is the sweetest person ever, to the crew at the Timepiece Ranch for making the experience so memorable, and to all the people who are involved in the Author Ready Group who have been so supportive and encouraging. It is because of all of you that I got my book finished.

With appreciation to all.

Love,

Paulette Ren

SPECIAL THANKS

IN WRITING THIS STORY there were so many more people that were involved in our lives that I didn't mention. They were all important in various ways and loved by me and my family. Many of these people played major roles, but I was trying to stick to certain events in our lives.

I would like to give thanks to my Mom and Dad, (Emma and Bruce), to my siblings, Frank, Mike, Renee, Roger, Chris, Cheryl, Kent, and Colleen. My In laws, Bob and Annie, Paul and Joann, Gary and Sue and the many aunts, uncles, and cousins, brought much help, love and concern and joy to us. They were a wonderful support system over the years.

Thanks to so many dear friends who talked to me when I needed to vent or helped in so many ways. Kathy and Paul, Jerene and Mike, Jeanne, Janice, Joanne and Cliff, Bev and Mike, Marie, and Dorothy. They were all there when I needed extra support. You all helped to save my sanity and look at what was important at that time. Your kindness and understanding were so appreciated.

I am here and feel so blessed. Antonio and I had a wonderful life in many ways despite all the obstacles that came our way. Thirty-three years was a long time to be together, but not long enough. I will cherish the wonderful memories for the rest of my life. So many stolen moments, but much to recollect in my aching heart. Thank you God for giving me the strength to continue with my life. It is because of all of you that I am writing this book.

I would like to thank Jessica Tanner for her endless help when needed, especially with all my computer needs. She knew how to do everything I didn't. I would have been lost without her. Also, I want to thank her daughter Sofia Tanner for her help in setting up my website. She knew just what I needed to make it happen. I'm so appreciative of all their work.

A SNEAK PEEK
INTO MY NEXT BOOK...

(Title to be determined)

When Antonio was sick in 1970'S, the doctor's said MS wasn't genetic.

So, I couldn't have been more shocked when one day in March of 2010, I received this phone call from my son Robert, who was thirty-four-years old.

"Hi, Mom, How are you?"

"I'm okay. What have you been up to?"

"Mom, I'm in the hospital. I have just been diagnosed with Multiple Sclerosis."

Releasing in 2024

www.ingramcontent.com/pod-product-compliance
Lightning Source LLC
Chambersburg PA
CBHW022059020426
42335CB00012B/749